Quacks and Cures:

Quack Doctors and Folk Healing of the Black Country

Kevin Goodman

Quacks and Cures:
Quack Doctors and Folk Healing of the Black Country
Published by
Bows, Blades and Battles Press
202 Ashenhurst Road,
Dudley,
West Midlands,
Dy1 2hz.

Copyright ©2017 Kevin Goodman
Kevin Goodman has asserted his right to be identified as the author
ISBN 978-0-9571377-2-1
First published 2017

Cover Illustration
W.E. Gladstone as a quack doctor selling remedies from his caravan; representing his advocacy of the Home Rule Bill in Parliament. Chromolithograph by T. Merry, (1889).The Wellcome Library. London.

http://bowsbladesandbattles.tripod.com

For Amelia Caitlin Rose
Who believes Daddy can make it better by kissing it.

ABOUT THE AUTHOR

Kevin Goodman is a historian, independent researcher, writer, historical interpreter and reenactor who specializes in the history of medicine and surgery. When not appearing around the country at various historical events demonstrating aspects of medicine and surgery throughout history, he is continually being outfoxed by his young daughter.

More details can be found at:
http://bowsbladesandbattles.tripod.com

By the same author:
Ouch! A History of Arrow Wound Treatment from Prehistory to the Nineteenth Century (2012)
ISBN 978-0-9571377-0-7

The Lords of Dudley Castle and the Welsh Wars of Edward I (2014)
ISBN 978-0-9571377-1-4

The Diggum Uppers: Body Snatching and Grave Robbing in the Black Country (2017)
ISBN 978-0-9571377-3-8

All are published by Bows, Blades & Battles Press

CONTENTS

Introduction: 1

Introduction

It cannot be denied: today we are fortunate.

When we fall ill we have access to a free National Health Service and, for the most part, easy access to doctors and medicines to cure us.

But imagine a time when there was no National Health Service and health care was restricted: dependent upon how much you could pay – if you could afford to pay.

Welcome to the Black Country of the past, where Quack Doctors, Charmers and Folk Cures held sway...

For readers who don't originate from the Black Country, the official Black Country History website[1] states that the Black Country is comprised of Dudley, Walsall, Sandwell and Wolverhampton and points out: *"It has no agreed borders and no two Black Country men or women will agree on where its starts or ends"*.

Author's Note

The name "the Black Country" for this industrial area of the West Midlands comes from Elihu Burritt's book *Walks in the Black Country and its Green Borderland* (1868), (Burit was the American Consular Agent to Birmingham), in which he described the view of the Black Country from the top of Dudley Castle:

"A writer of a military turn of fancy might say that it was the sublimest battle-scene ever enacted on earth . . . There was an embattled amphitheatre of twenty miles span ridged to the purple clouds. Planted at artillery intervals on this encircling ridge, and at musket-shot spaces in the dark valley between, a thousand batteries, mounted with huge ordnance, white at the mouth with the fury of the bombardment, were pouring their cross-fires of shot and shell into the cloud-works of the lower heavens. Wolverhampton, on the extreme left, stood by her black

---

[1] http://blackcountryhistory.org/places

mortars which shot their red volleys into the night. Coseley and Bilston and Wednesbury replied bomb for bomb, and set the clouds on fire above with their lighted matches. Dudley, Oldbury, Albion, and Smethwick, on the right, plied their heavy breachers at the iron-works on the other side; while West Bromwich and distant Walsall showed that their men were standing as bravely to their guns, and that their guns were charged to the muzzle with the grape and canister of the mine. The canals twisting and crossing through the field of battle, showed by patches in the light like bleeding veins."

Authors Note:

I really shouldn't have to say this but:

Do not try any of the remedies or cures contained within this book. They are purely for historical interest and not intended for use. They could prove harmful if used. The author cannot be held responsible in such cases.

In other words:

If yow'm saft enough to try 'em, dow cum blaertin' to me when yow'm took bad!

(Translation: If you are silly enough to try them don't come crying to me when you fall ill!)

1) THE QUACK DOCTORS

The image of the Quack Doctor we have today is very much influenced by the American "Snake Oil Salesman" (via Saturday and Sunday afternoon cowboy films): a conman who knowingly sells fraudulent medicines and then hotfoots it out of town before he is tarred and feathered, or lynched, by his duped victims.

However, the reality in the Black Country was somewhat different.

The definition of a Quack Doctor according to the Oxford English Dictionary is *"A person who dishonestly claims to have special knowledge and skill in some field; typically medicine"*. The name is derived from the phrase *Quacksalver*, which comes from the Dutch *kwakzalver* meaning a *"hawker of salve"*, in the medieval period *Quack* meant "shouting". Up until the early part of the twentieth century it would have been difficult to visit a Black Country market and not encounter a number of these Quacks announcing the healing virtues of their particular cures at the top of their voices.

These quack remedies, which included emetics (which caused vomiting); laxatives (increased bowel movements) and diuretics (increased urination), frequently contained no effective curative ingredients whatsoever. Some contained substances such as alcohol and opium - addictive qualities which would have enticed buyers to return, while some contained toxic ingredients such as mercury and arsenic (Porter 2003).

However, many Quacks were rarely run out of town, (or given the Black Country equivalent of tar and feathering: throwing them in the canal), and had permanent pitches at Black Country markets and regular customers.

As to why people resorted to such Quacks and their remedies, there are a number of reasons (Porter 2003):

Cost: Prior to 1948 and the establishment of the National Health Service, free healthcare was limited. Free treatment was sometimes available from Voluntary Hospitals, (such as the Dudley Dispensary, established in 1862 and the Stourbridge Dispensary established in the 1830's), which were established by charities, and funded via charitable donations. However these were for the benefit of the *'deserving poor'*, who, according to Victorian values, were respectable working-class people who had fallen on hard times because of sickness. The sick and destitute, (*"the undeserving poor"*), were regarded as being responsible for their own misfortunes, (alcoholics, unmarried mothers, beggars, unemployed and unemployed parents with large families), and had no alternative but to seek admission into a workhouse which had their own infirmaries where residents could be treated. For working men who could afford it under the National Insurance Act (1911), a small amount was deducted from their weekly wages, to which were added contributions from the employer and the government. In return the workman was entitled to medical care (as well as retirement and unemployment benefits) although not necessarily to the drugs prescribed, which had to be paid for, however, their families and women and children were not covered. Local chemist shops also provided a source of treatment for a fee. As a result some people could not afford, or did not qualify for, treatment and had no alternative to the treatments offered by Quack Doctors.

Causal Beliefs: Today it is accepted that illness can be caused by germs, viruses, genetic conditions and/or lifestyle. Up until the late nineteenth century it was still accepted that illness was the result of an imbalance in the four humours, (blood, phlegm, yellow bile and black bile), a theory that originated with the ancient Greek physician Hippocrates (c.480BC-c.370BC). The imbalance of the humours resulted from lifestyle (diet, alcohol intake, physical activity, moral behaviour) and the impact of miasma: poisoned air which could be breathed in or absorbed through a person's skin, (diseases including cholera, typhus, small pox and the bubonic plague were all attributed to miasma). From the 1860's with the discovery of bacteria by Louis Pasteur (1822-1895) and the discovery by Robert Koch (1843-1910) of the Tuberculosis bacillus in 1876 and Anthrax Bacillus in 1882, germ theory became accepted. However, it was not accepted by all: Florence Nightingale (1820-1910) was initially opposed to it. As a result, less educated people may have been wary of accepting such novel ideas, preferring the more familiar causal beliefs propagated by the Quacks.

Regression fallacy: Certain conditions, such as warts and the common cold, almost always improve over time. In the past, prior to the widespread understanding of the impact of illnesses and their effects, patients may have associated the usage of quack treatments with recovery, when recovery was, in fact, inevitable.

Placebo effect: Medicines or treatments which are known to have no pharmacological effect on a disease can still affect a person's perception of their illness, and this belief can have a therapeutic effect, causing the patient's condition to improve.

Conspiracy theories: Conspiracy theories, such as the controversy over the Measles, Mumps and Rubella (MMR) vaccine (Poland 2011; Mnookin 2012; Bliss 2014) are not a modern phenomenon. There were concerns when widespread smallpox vaccination was introduced in the nineteenth century. It was introduced following Edward Jenner's cowpox experiments, in which he demonstrated that he could protect a child from smallpox if he infected it with pus from a cowpox blister. Despite its efficacy it was a novel idea that went against the medical philosophy of the day, (that small pox was caused by miasma: poisonous matter in the atmosphere). It was met with immediate public criticism from physicians who adhered to the medical beliefs of the time and the church who objected due to their belief that the vaccine was unchristian because it came from an animal. For example, on May 21st 1881, the *London Brief News and Opinion* reported that most of the schools in Dudley and the Black Country were closed to prevent children being vaccinated against small pox. This stemmed from the belief that William Gladstone, the Prime Minister, was trying to control population growth through killing off children through vaccinations.

All the Black Country markets had Quack Doctors. The Black

Country poet Ben Boucher (1769-1851) observed in his 1827 poem "Lines on Dudley Market":

> *"Kash from Walsall kills the worms*
> *Judas brings a salve for corns*
> *Mind these men or you'll be bitten*
> *Black Jack's wife brings salve from Tipton"*

Walter White in his book "*All round the Wrekin*" (1860) describes a visit to Dudley on Market Day and the quack doctors he found there:

"The doctors find it worthwhile to appear and make proclamation of their skill, and show their remedies. One, who had bottled up a worm nearly as long as a boa constrictor, harangued the multitude with an assumption of scientific knowledge enough to put the whole College of Physicians to shame; "I am no M.D.," he cried, "and I'm not ashamed to own it. I'm something better, for I can cure them as want to be cured, without charging a guinea for it. For five-and-twenty years have I stood in Dudley-market, curing no end o'people, and shan't fret if they don't put up a statue to my memory when I'm dead. Where's any o'your regular M.D.'s as can say the same? If there's any of ye have got anything the matter, you've only got to try my herbal pills, grown from the homogeneous mass of the earth, and you'll find 'em expel, eradicate, and destroy, all the sluggish phlegm and slime which undermine and injure the principles of health. My herbal pills will set ye straight and sound; if you haven't tried 'em, just look at those anatomical specimens of worms, look at those jars of coloured liquors, showing the state of your juices all true to morbid nature, and you'll see the corrupt and dangerous state of your insides" (p249-50).

And also those on Walsall market:

"…strangest of all was the sight of perhaps a dozen stalls scattered among the others, exhibiting an array of glass jars and bullets , some filled with bright yellow liquid, some with various kinds of worms, some with a green substance looking like a preparation of cabbage leaves, some with bullets. By each stood a glib tongued orator, vociferating the virtues of his vegetable medicines, extolling the efficacy of his pills (which I had taken for bullets) and pointing to the ghastly

exhibition of worms as the consequence of neglect of his warnings and recommendations. These orators are the doctors of the neighbourhood, consulted by miners, labourers and artisans. I saw one poor woman asking advice for her infant son in arms and watched the result. The doctor prescribed pills and put three of the bullets in a box, with instructions to administer half a one at intervals dissolved in sugared water" (p249).

According to Freeman (1931) Bilston Market had a number of regular Quack Doctors in the early part of the twentieth century:

Dr. Nathaniel Catlin. Known as *"Old Texas"* he wore a variety of clothe from the American West: a broad sombrero hat, a Stetson, a ten gallon hat, a bear skin coat, (which he insisted was fashioned from the hide of a grizzly bear he had shot between the eyes with his last bullet during a perilous expedition into the Rocky Mountains), or buckskin clothes. He spoke with an American accent and told tales of his life in the American West. He claimed to be a native of Chicago and that his father was a solicitor there. Although he had trained for the medical profession he had failed to qualify and was never able to practice, although he had served in the American navy for four years as an assistant surgeon. He also claimed George Catlin (1796-1872) the American adventurer, artist and author was his uncle and that he was a close friend of Buffalo Bill and other noted frontiersmen. One tale he told about his life on the prairie was how he was riding alone one day and his horse threw him, breaking both his legs. He lay there for many hours but when no help arrived and he was forced to perform first aid upon himself, then to crawl a long distance to reach the nearest house where he obtained skilled help. Described as being haughty and contemptuous of the other Quacks on the market, his stall was crowded with herbs he claimed had been gathered in the prairie wilds by Native American women he also carried a staff from which herbs hung. A sign on his stall read *"Dr.Catlin, Vendor of secret Indian cures for all ailments"* and he claimed he could cure anything from gout to a fractured skull. About his herbs he talked eloquently, pouring out a string of botanical terms. His sharp and witty tongue drew the crowds to him and into verbal duels with his rival "Doctor

Dick" in which the latter did not always emerge triumphant. After many years of successful business in the market place, he quarrelled with the market authorities and contemptuously declared he would never show his face there again. After this he opened a herb shop in Bilston High Street; at the front of his shop was a stall where he sold *"Buffalo Bill Candy"*.

Doctor Dick. Dicky Hill or, as he preferred to be called, *"Dr. Dick"*, started out as an ironworker, but drifted onto the market where his ready wit, his gift for good natured teasing and his talent for storytelling made him an amusing entertainer, allowing him to secure many customers for his remedies. In his early days on the market he dressed as a clown and never failed to entertain his audience. He was extremely versatile - to draw in a crowd of customers and hold it: he would sing songs; tell tales; reel doggerels and tell jokes. He would also draw his crowd with a burst of noise from his instruments: a blast from his horn; a tattoo on his kettle drum; a tune on his windy bagpipes and the ringing of a triangle.

He would then commence business with a challenging shout: *"Leave all the other fools and come to me!"* This would result in a battle of banter with his rivals which he did not always win, (he said of Catlin *"The nearest Old Tex has been to a redskin is when he's eating a tomato!"*). However: he always won his crowd if he sometimes lost the laugh to his rivals. His opening rhyme was:

"I'm Dr.Dick.
Who cures quick,
I have a pill,
Cures every ill."

To which he added: *"It will cure bad temper and empty pockets: who'll try it?"*

This was usually followed with a yarn in which he would reel off a long list of miraculous cures:

- *"Did I ever tell you,"* he would ask *"How I took a man's leg off, and put it on again in five minutes?"* (Following calls of disbelief, he would relate how he repaired a collier's wooden leg).

- *"Why, only last week, my pills cured a little girl of consumption. The doctor told her, her left lung had gone, and then that the right one had gone also. So when I took her in hand she'd got no lungs at all. Then after the first box of pills, her left lung came back, and then her right lung came back as well. Did I hear somebody laugh!?! You don't believe it !?! You can please yourself! But perhaps when you've got no lungs you'll be glad to come to Dr. Dick to try his pills".*

- *"Now all you hard working folks come here! And I'll tell you how to do without hard work!!"* (The secret was to take a box of his pills which were guaranteed to work off back ache and cure wooden legs).

- Of himself he used to say: *"In my fool's days I worked hard enough. It only took one donkey to draw me out of the works, but a dozen wouldn't take me back again!"*

He also sold sarsaparilla, (a sweet soft drink thought to have many medicinal properties and was drunk as a curative tonic), claiming it was as miraculous as his pills. Holding up a glass he would say: *"That's the stuff to put new life into you! Do you more good that a glass of old* [beer]. *It'll make old men jump like a pony and as for appetite you'll want a truss of hay".*

Occasionally he went too far. One day he was freely giving away several glasses of his tonic and offered one to a well dressed stranger - who politely declined it. Dick was piqued and said: *"Have it, it won't poison thee!"*

"No thank you, I don't want it." said the stranger.

"You have to have it." replied Dick

"No, I shall not!" insisted the stranger

"I'll make thee! There!" And with that, Dick threw the sarsaparilla into the man's face.

The stranger gripped one of the legs on Dick's stall and snapped it off then swung it - smashing up Dick's stall - boxes of his lozenges, pills and medicines were smashed and scattered. Dick fell upon the other man - they struggled and fought - the pair rolling on the ground several times. The verdict was that Dick's tongue was a better weapon than his fists.

For some years he rode to market on a cart pulled by a donkey while playing a drum. One day he announced that his customers were going to show their gratitude by purchasing for him a new van and on the following Monday he would ride into the market in triumph drawn by the finest pair of steeds in the town and led by a famous brass band. That Monday his entrance drew a crowd: he rode in on an old furniture van pulled by a donkey, while his own ambled behind. On the van, (which he had also repaired and ornamented), he had painted the word: "*Antilocopharmacutagoria*". In front of him walked four very wheezy bandsmen while Dick sat on the driver's seat banging away at a triangle and kettle drum while a musician followed behind playing a mournful accompaniment upon a big drum.

He travelled around the local markets including Dudley and Wolverhampton. When he visited Wolverhampton market to sell his cures he would leave his donkey and van at the Star and Garter Inn. Sometimes he would linger into the late hours drinking and entertaining his fellow imbibers. On one occasion a stranger was annoyed because he had missed the last train to Bilston. In his best manner, Dick replied: "*My carriage will be at the door presently and I shall be delighted to give the gentleman a lift*". The offer was gratefully accepted and the stranger, relieved, enjoyed the entertainment. Come the early hours, Dick called out "*Bring my carriage round please*"; with a grin the stable man brought around the ramshackle vehicle. "*I'll arrange the seats and cushions*" said Dick, nipping off to rearrange his bottles and boxes to make an extra seat. When he returned he announced "*Now, Sir, my carriage is at your service*". However, the stranger had no sense of humour and when he saw his carriage, abused Dick for his deception and refused to accompany him.

However, he fell afoul of the local doctors: he would place M.D. (Medical Doctor) after his name and following complaints the Medical Association initiated legal proceedings against him. When brought before the magistrate charged with using the title of Medical Doctor, he denied it. *"What then does M.D. mean?"* asked the magistrate. He replied: *"Oh that means 'Merry Dick' and it means 'Money Down'. Mine's a ready money business."* The magistrate was not amused and he had to drop the letters and pay a fine.

The Turner Brothers. These were regarded as the elite among the Black Country Quacks. For many years they had a large lock up stall in the front market of Bilston. They were well versed in anatomy, using life sized diagrams of the human body and intricate models of the internal organs which they took to pieces to the amazement of the gaping crowd. Both resented the title of *"Quack"* claiming to have a better knowledge of the healing arts than most doctors. They took themselves very seriously and rarely tried to amuse. While one lectured the other had charge of the consulting room into which there was always a stream of patients.

Old Sarsaparilla. Mr. Appleby *"The Sarsaparilla Man"* would repeat endlessly his well known cry: *"Sarsaparilla: The Great Blood Purifier, half-penny and a penny a glass"*. He had a stream of customers every week for a dose to remedy the effects of their excesses. Unfortunately, due to his weak and squeaky voice and nervous tics, he was the victim of mischievous boys who would wait until his attention was diverted then turn on the tap of his sarsaparilla tanks and run away.

Cough Drops. He was a tall man, thin and slow and heavy of speech, he sold herbal sweets and powders. He would call out his wares in rhyme. A familiar one was:

> *"For backache, headache, toothache*
> *I've a cure for all on the stall*
> *Come all who suffer*
> *And try it*
> *And if I don't cure you one and all*
> *You'd be very foolish to buy it."*

Other Quacks on Bilston market included a tall Afro-Caribbean man clad in an ill-fitting evening dress suit and claimed to have cured all the crowned heads in Europe with his wonderful snuff and a man in a worn out carriage who wore a non-descript military uniform and claimed to have sold his magic salve in every known part of the world.

During the 1930's Quacks were regular visitors to Wednesbury Market (see Humphries: *"It seems like yesterday"*). One claimed to be a descendent of a Native American Indian chief: dressed in a leather coat with an Indian brave painted on the back he sold Rattlesnake Oil. He would extol the remarkable healing properties of the oil. After much convincing patter, describing how to take the oil by mouth, or by rubbing it in, (depending on the particular affliction), he would offer small quantities of rare medicine for sale. However, he would always explain that due to the difficulty of extracting the oil his supply was very limited. He always sold out. One Quack, a gentleman of colour, sold extract of Mandrake root and he had his own method of securing the audience's sympathy and attention. In the crowd a heckler would always appear and proceed to shout disparagingly about the medicine, making offensive comments about the colour of the Quack's skin and other derogatory comments, (all of which had been previously agreed upon by the Quack and the heckler). This attack would arouse sympathy for the Quack and after a while members of the crowd would be leaping to his defence – and purchasing bottles of his remedy. One Quack prepared his "body cleansing" pills in a public house near the High Bullen. The pills consisted of very small bits of Sunlight soap rolled into pills in flour on the pub table.

Walsall market was home to a variety of Quack Doctors and their remedies until the mid-twentieth century:

"Quack doctors, and they used to descend in a swarm in Walsall Market and they were some of the rummest characters you ever met. Some were quite genuine in their own way. There used to be a herbalist, I remember, one of the genuine ones, I think he was a Pole, his name was Wasser and he had a little herbalist shop at the end of Goodall Street. And I can see the shop now, it really

was like a house window, I think it was a house and he had turned the front room into a shop. And hanging up on the window were all sorts of quasi-medical junk including a couple of cork legs. One of those heads you used to see, all marked out in squares[2], I forget what they call the practice, telling your fortune and everything, but he had one of those in the window and a display of trusses all over the place hanging up on each side of the window like a festoon. The prize display item was a model of the electric chair from Sing Sing. He claimed it was a true model of the Sing Sing chair and he used to bring this out into the market on a Saturday night and perch it on a tall box from which he used to pontificate to the crowd, he used to sell herbs and medicines all sorts and herbs that would cure every ruddy complaint under the sun. He did a marvelous trade and would extract a tooth for you for a tanner[3]. I never saw him actually do it I have stood around for hours hoping someone would want a tooth out. But I am assured by many contenders at the time that when he had successfully taken a tooth out for someone, which he did most adroitly, and I expect painfully, when he'd done it, he used to blow a trumpet you know and then extract the tanner from the bloke who would get away as fast as he could to get away from the admiring crowd. He was only one of the patent medicine wallahs there, there were several, every Saturday there were several, they used to have little pots of this and boxes of that but it was their spieling that used to fascinate me as a boy. The common spiel was how degenerate the man of the day had got and that the herbs he sold restored virility ... I always remember one, a particularly villainous character he was, who posed as being a struck off doctor and he told a marvellous story about the pills he sold that would cure any female ailment under the sun you know.

"I think mostly I have been told by people who knew the business a bit, most of them were soft soap and bitter aloes rolled into pills and then dusted with something. Anyway he used to get a very big crowd around him and it used to be most fascinating to watch the crowd, most of them would take this yarn in and when he'd finished he used to start to sell. First of all his famous virility pills and

---

[2] A phrenology head: Phrenology was the detailed study of the shape and size of the cranium as an indication of character and mental abilities

[3] Tanner: Sixpence equal to 2 ½ pence.

they'd go like hot cakes at a tanner a box…"

"There were several men like him about the market in those days all on the same racket selling medicines, some of them weren't medicines. I was assured by a bloke that had seen it done. One of the chaps, selling a marvelous cure all ointment that would fix anything under the sun, he used to buy a pound of lard and an old kitchen knife and he'd slap the lard into little boxes and put the lids on…

"There was one chap from Birmingham by the name of Doctor Barry; He wasn't a doctor really just a market trader. He used to sell cold cures stuff. You'd put a few drops on your handkerchief and you'd just take a good breath and that cleared your head. You see, it did clear your head because it was sort of pure carbolic stuff . . . it was like pure disinfectant, and he used to put a drop of this on somebody's handkerchief, 'smell that my love', 'cause it used to knock your head off nearly you see. Then he used to charge them half a crown for a little bottle of this, which was the pure stuff mixed with a drop of water" (p8-9 Walsall Local History Centre 1992).

Some Quack Doctors travelled from door to door: Old Michael was a former handyman who preferred to sell his salves and lotions from door to door. He had a way of securing himself a large number of patients: he would knock on a door, then peeping into the house would say:

"Mrs you're not looking so well today."

The answer was often: *"No I'm feeling quite well"*

"No you aren't. I can see it. Now if you take this …"

"But I don't have anything to do with quacks?"

"I'm not a quack, I go about to do people good. If you keep this bottle I shall charge you only half the price now and if it does you good you can pay the rest when I come again in a week."

Going into house he had previously visited he would say: *"Ah, I can see you are better, I can tell you are"* usually with a request for the balance.

To patients he would say: *"You can take the medicine with a little drop of rum"*. Sometimes the customers would say:*"But I don't like rum"*. Then he would reply *"Then it will do just as well with gin, or in a cup of tea."*

The local priest was concerned about Michael's calling and often remarked: *"Be careful Michael, or I'm afraid you'll get into trouble yet"*.

'*Never fear, father, if the physic I give them does then no good, it will do them no harm"* was his reply. (Freeman 1931).

Some areas had their own particular quack cures: Darlaston had a woman known for her two ointments: *"Draw it out"* for drawing boils and carbuncles and *"Heal it up"* for healing cuts and sores; at Hurst Hill, a woman prepared sticking plasters for drawing boils – the ingredients of the mixture were never divulged – although they were so effective it was said they could draw the inside out of a brick; at Old Hill cuts, grazes and festering wounds were treated with Page's ointment, a gritty yellow mixture made locally and sold in small stone jars and at Brierley Hill "Blue Oils" could be obtained to cure whooping cough, (Brimble 1986).

A number of Acts between 1938 and 1941 (the Food and Drugs Act 1938; the Cancer Act 1939; the Pharmacy and Medicines Act 1941) effectively outlawed Quacks and the open sale of their remedies and the start of the National Health Service in 1948 where medicine was available for free put an end to them.

However that is not to say medicines sold legitimately were any safer.

2 PATENT MEDICINES

A patent medicine, was a commercial medicine, sold over the counter by many chemists and did not require a Doctor's prescription. They were frequently heavily advertised as being medical panaceas (cure alls) or - at the very least - a treatment for a large number of diseases. They emphasised exotic ingredients and were accompanied by endorsements from purported experts and/or celebrities, (which may or may have not been true). Many, especially those advertised as being "infant soothers", contained opium and alcohol.

There were many patent medicines available for soothing infants: *Dalby's Carminative, Daffy's Elixir, Atkinson's Infants' Preservative, Mrs. Winslow's Soothing Syrup , Mother's Quietness,* and *Street's Infants' Quietness.* The most popular patent medicine in the Black Country was *"Godfrey's Cordial"*, a mixture of opium, wine and treacle, known as "Comfort," and used when the mother wished to work or keep her children quiet.

An advertisement for Godfrey's Cordial in the *Wolverhampton Chronicle and Staffordshire Advertiser* (17th November 1830) stated:

"GODFREY'S CORDIAL"
The genuine GODFREY'S CORDIAL is a Medicine so well known, and so efficacious in most of the complaints incidental to young children"

In their investigations which concluded with the Children's Employment Commission Reports of 1842-3 inspectors had concerns about its use. They described the case of Priscilla Hatton, aged 10 years, of Stourbridge who looked after her younger sister while her parents were at work:

"[Priscilla] *works at home at nursing: the child is one month old. Is considered a good nurse by her mother; the child is a good child, "but it squeaks a*

THE GRAND MEDICINE OF THE DAY!

SQUIRE KNIGHT'S

CELEBRATED

PURIFYING FAMILY PILLS.

These celebrated Pills have for the last HUNDRED YEARS proved very superior to every other Medicine offered to the Public in the cure of Indigestion, Bilious Complaints, Loss of Appetite, Sick Headache, Giddiness in the Head, Pain and Fulness after Meals, Wind, Heartburn, Lowness of Spirits, Piles, Worms, Shortness of Breath, Nervous Disease, Cramps, Spasms, Fevers, Affections of the Liver, Dimness of Sight, Pains in the Stomach and Bowels, Eruptions of the Skin, &c., &c.

TESTIMONIALS.

Mrs. Job Stephens, of Woodside, Dudley, was perfectly cured of Wind and Spasms, of one year's duration, by taking these celebrated Pills.

Amelia Griffiths, of Mostyn, was cured of nine years' affliction of Indigestion by taking two boxes of these Pills.

Joseph Wagstaff, of Dudley Port, was afflicted with a severe Pain in his Side for four years, but was cured before he had taken two boxes of these Pills.

Mrs. Davis, of Kingswinford, was cured of constant Costiveness, Pains in the Bowels, and Giddiness in the Head, by taking these Pills.

Susannah Brewster, Herbert Street, Wolverhampton, was cured of a very bad Liver Complaint by taking "Squire Knight's Purifying Pills."

Henry McKay, Woodside, Dudley, has proved these Pills to be the best for Indigestion, Wind, Heartburn, and a Disordered Stomach.

Mrs. Beard, High Street, Bradley, was cured of a very serious Outbreak, arising from Impurities in the Blood, besides relieving a Congested Liver, and acting upon the Stomach and Bowels.

PREPARED BY

C. F. G. CLARK & SON,

(SUCCESSORS TO SQUIRE KNIGHT),

CHEMISTS, MARKET PLACE, DUDLEY.

Above: A Nineteenth Century advertisement for *Squire Knight's Celebrated Purifying Pills* which cured a variety of ailments according to testimonials from satisfied customers from around the Black Country and were available from a number of reputable chemists

little sometimes when her wants tittee": mother gives it a tea-spoonful of Godfrey's Cordial, about three times a-day; sometimes she (witness) gives the child a teaspoonful of Godfrey's Cordial when mother's out, and the child is noisy and restless; always knows where to find the Godfrey's Cordial; takes a little herself sometimes, because it's nice; it makes her go to sleep too as well as the child, and it's very nice." (p.520 *Report and Appendices of the Children's Employment Commission* 1843).

In the report Mr. Cooper, a surgeon of Bilston, stated:

"The chief evil which they have to endure is, that when very young their mothers injure them by quackery, and give opiates, such as Godfrey's Cordial, which is a mixture of treacle and opium. Many deaths are caused by quack medicines. Medical men seldom see the children until they are benumbed and stupified with opiates." (p.68 *The Condition And Treatment Of The Children Employed In The Mines And Collieries Of The United Kingdom* 1842).

However in the same report a respectable Dudley Chemist states he made twenty gallons of "comfort" in a year and that there were chemists near the market place who made far more.

Epidemics brought with them an increase in patent cures. During the Cholera epidemic of 1832 local newspapers contained a number of advertisements for cures and remedies of dubious quality and reliability:

The Wolverhampton Chronicle 23rd November 1831:

"Cholera Morbus"

"Medical practitioners being agreed in the recommendation of warm bathing in Cholera Morbus. Mr. Coleman calls the attention of the public to MR.WHITLAW'S PATENT MEDICATED VAPOUR BATH, *as being far superior to any other mode of bathing , and especially under the attack of this dreadful disease, as has been proved by Dr. Fairbanks , of Bahia, Mr. Owen, of Calcutta, as well as by various practitioners in South Carolina.*

Should the Asiatic Cholera appear in this neighbourhood, Mr. Coleman purposes to appropriate one or more Baths, as occasion may require, for the gratuitous use of the poor.

Mr. Coleman continues to treat with the greatest success, the following diseases by means of the Medical Vapour Bath (in conjunction with other remedies,) Rheumatism, Gout, Asthma, Scrofula, Cancerous tumour sin their incipient stage, Cutaneous Diseases, Liver Complaints, Debility, and all disorders arising from derangement of the Digestive Organs.

Portable baths applicable to those cases where the patient is confined either to bed or room."

The *Staffordshire Advertiser* 15th September 1832:
"Important Discovery"

"Abraham's Cholericus. This invaluable remedy for CHOLERA, DIARRHŒA, and DYSENTERY, has been discovered by C.J. ABRAHAM, Chemist and has given relief to thousands of persons suffering from these dreadful disorders. In different parts of England its virtue has been fully proved, and many cases of malignant cholera have yielded to its astonishing powers. The flattering testimonials received by the proprietor, from gentlemen of the highest respectability, both in and out of the profession. Induce him to offer it to the public as a safe and   effectual remedy for each of the above-named diseases, in their most malignant form. Let the patients use it immediately, and they may confidently rely on its efficacy.

This powerful medicine, administered according to the simple directions which accompany each bottle, may be taken with the best effect, and perfect safety, by patients in the lowest state of debility, and even by infants of the most tender years, when properly diluted. It is not depending on astringency for its effects, it is a simple but chemical remedy, which will be found to neutralize and remove the deleterious gases , which accumulate in the stomach, bowels, &c., and produce such direful effects.

The *Wolverhampton Chronicle* October 10th 1832:
"MORISON'S UNIVERSAL VEGETABLE MEDICINE"
Cure of four Persons in one Family of the Cholera.
To Mr. Morison.
DEAR SIR. *As a complete testimony of the power of the "Universal Medicines" over the Cholera, I hereby transmit to you from the extraordinary circumstances of four individuals in this house, who have been all cured, by them alone, of this*

dreadful malady which is sending hundreds to their graves all around us, My brother, about the 28th July, was taken ill; but, paying little attention to it at the time, the symptoms of the disorder became so alarming that medical aid was resorted to. At that time he was awfully cramped in the lower parts of the stomach and bowels; extremely relaxed, so that every thing passed through him immediately, or was thrown up with most violent retching; his countenance indicated a speedy dissolution, and the cry was "he is dying." The medical gentlemen used the various methods in common practice in cholera (which were the decided opinion of the complaint), such as blisters, mustard plasters, and other treatments, the best they know of; but all in vain, for they said nothing but a miracle can save him, and gave him up in despair. In this extremity the fame of the "Universal Medicines" having cured many patients in this dreadful malady, we were induced to apply to Mr.T.Round of Tipton, sub-agent under your general Stafford agent. Mr. Mason of West Bromwich, and purchased some pills; and his reasoning with me and my friends, on the propriety of giving large doses, in order to meet the virulence of the case with immediate and full force, inspired us with such confidence, that we acted promptly to his advice , and before 30 pills of No.2 were administered , we observed an evident change for the better, and, to cut my story short, to the astonishment of all around us , he recovered, and is now, thank the Almighty and you, the happy instrument, in full health. Having been more particular in this first case, I need but shortly add that three more of the family, my father, my sister, and another brother, were all similarly attacked, the two former of whom flew immediately to the same means, and were soon recovered; but my brother, not having the same courage, resisted, and sunk past all hope of relief; when, at length, he called me to his bed, and said, "I feel I am dying; "I replied, "Not so, If you take Morison's Pills.". He then rallied, and consented, and the result was, he is as hearty and well as the rest. For the good of the suffering world at this dread time of pestilence, you are at full liberty to give publicity to this my plain unvarnished tale of facts; and may the God of Heaven bless you, and all concerned in this great work of merit, is the ardent prayer of, dear Sir (in behalf of all our family,) your humble servant,

JAMES FERIDAY

Workhouse Lane, Tipton, Staffordshire,
10th September , 1832."

Eventually, with the introduction of various acts surrounding medicines, patent medicines were brought under control. However a number of familiar brands dating from the era of the patent medicine still exist, but their ingredients have changed and the claims regarding their benefits have been revised. These include: Andrew's Liver Salts; Phillips' Milk of Magnesia and Vicks Vapour Rub. Other existing products which were once marketed as patent medicines include: Bovril; Coca Cola; Tonic Water; Pepsi Cola and 7 up.

3 CHARMERS

It was not only Quacks and chemists who were the purveyors of dubious cures. As with the Quacks, lack of access to medical care due to cost meant that Charmers or Folk Healers, (people who cured through enchantments and spells), were also frequently consulted. Often, these men and women were people of high regard in their communities, the women frequently being called upon to help pregnant women give birth or to lay out (prepare) the deceased for burial.

In the 1820's an old woman living in the yard of the "Hen and Chickens" public house, Dudley St., Wolverhampton did a "roaring" trade in charming warts, curing black eyes and treating children with the "chin cough" (whooping cough[4]) and measles[5] (Poole 1875). Freeman (1931) describes an old woman who lived within a mile of Bilston Town Hall who was professed to charm away warts and toothache and had many customers. The most famous of the Black Country Charmers was Theophilus "Elijah" Dunn from Bumble Hole, Netherton also known as *Devil Dunn"* or the *"Dudley Devil"*.

Apart from being a charmer and healer he was also a tracer of lost property and fortune teller. Far from being ignorant, he was well educated and well acquainted with the works of famous astrologers and could also cast horoscopes. Despite local people believing he had dealings with the devil, he drew clients from Worcester, Stafford, London and Scotland, however he would charge according to the

---

[4] Whooping Cough: A highly contagious bacterial disease, while the symptoms are similar to the common cold it is characterised by a high-pitched whoop sound or gasp as the person breathes in following a fit of coughing. Known in the Black Country as the "Chin Cough".

[5] Measles is a highly infectious viral illness characterised by a red-brown blotchy rash that can lead to serious complications.

circumstance of his customer.

According to Palmer (2007) Dunn was asked, in the 1840's, by a Dudley school master as to what life would be like two hundred years in the future. He is reputed to have prophesised:

"So quickly in time will they travel
That there'll be no here or there
They'll pass by the moon in the bullet
And live on cold cloud and hot air".

In 1850 the famed pugilist (bare knuckle boxer) William Perry, "The Tipton Slasher" (1819-1881) consulted Dunn with regard to what the future held for him. Dunn replied:

"Slasher, yow'll stop as yow started,
Yow'll get all yow gid in one goo.
Yow and yer pub will be parted
Tom Little will mek it cum true"

"Tom Little" is thought to be the pugilist Tom Sayers (1826-1865). The Slasher lost to Sayers in 1857 and was left penniless since he had sold the public house he owned and all his possessions in order to back himself to win.

Dunn's nickname *"Elijah"* was given to any Black Country man who had the power of prophecy, (after the biblical prophet Elijah).

When recovering stolen articles, after he had received his fee from the client, he would ask a number of probing questions concerning the people living in the house and visitors: learning all he could about the case. He would give instructions, including a charm, on how to act if the property was not returned within a set time. The news of the visit to the Devil soon spread, along with a hint that the thief would be soon be revealed. The thief – if he or she was just as superstitious – would return the goods without his or her identity becoming known. However, this tactic was not always successful at scaring hardened criminals and his charms would be ignored.

Hackwood (1924) records one of Dunn's charms for toothache: the sufferer was to take a piece of paper and write on it:

> *"Peter...sat...at the gate of Jerusalem...Jesus passed by...and said...What aileth thee, Peter?...Peter said...unto Jesus...my teeth ache...and are sore...I am unable...to stand or walk...Jesus said...rise and walk, Peter...In the name...of the father...son...and Holy Ghost...He that puts faith...in these words I now speak..his teeth shall never ache."*

The charm was to be worn close to the sufferer's body. The charge for it was one shilling.

After some successful years, his reputation began to wane and his trade declined, he went to live at Dudley Port and carried on fortune telling. He committed suicide by hanging, at the age of 60, in 1851. He was buried in St. Andrew's churchyard, Netherton, where, according to legend, for many years his gravestone was always scrubbed. This was a service wives and mothers did for their departed but Dunn had no close relatives and no one ever saw it being scrubbed.

Folk Cures

Black Country Charmers, or Healers, frequently utilised folk cures or remedies, which were handed down from generation to generation, to cure the illnesses which plagued their customers:

Ague (shivering fit) *and Fever:* Eat a stew made from rooks feet and dock leaves.

Asthma: Eat raw carrots.

Bed Wetting: Eat the internal organs of a mouse fried.

Bee Stings: Rub a "blue bag" on it. (A blue bag, which contained synthetic ultramarine and baking soda was used on washing days to whiten white clothes).

Black eyes and bruises: Apply a poultice of bruised carrots and plant resin.

Boils:

-Place a hot bread poultice over it.

-Place soap mixed with sugar over the boil.

-Place a bottle or glass that had been warmed over a flame over the boil. This created a vacuum which would draw the boil. This has its origins in the practice of "cupping" which dates back to the Romans.

Bumps to the head:

-Apply butter.

-Apply vinegar and brown paper.

Bunions: Take a small piece of raw beef and press it onto the bunion for seven hours then bury it. As the meat decayed the bunion would disappear.

Chilblains:

-Two strong boys held the afflicted person while a third thrashed his foot with a handful of holly.

-Rub a raw onion on the feet.

-Soak the feet in a chamber pot full of stale human urine or rub the urine on the feet.

Choke Damp (The result of having been choked by gas in mines): Remove a sod of earth from the ground and place the mouth of the sufferer over the hole. The drawing action of the earth would cause the noxious gases to leave the patient.

Colds: To ward off a cold smell the sweat from a worn sock.

Corns (Calluses on the feet caused by excessive pressure on the skin, usually caused by poorly fitting shoes):

-Wet them nine mornings in succession with one's own fasting spittle.

-Take small piece of raw beef and press it onto the corn for seven hours then bury it. As the meat decayed the corn would disappear.

Coughs:

-Rub Goose fat on chest and back and wrap brown paper over the chest and back and leave it for three days.

-Swallow mustard and melted butter or apply the mixture to the chest and cover with brown paper.

-Take a mixture of butter, sugar and vinegar.

-Put Demerara sugar between two slices of turnip and swallow a tablespoon of the resulting juice three times a day.

-Eat burnt toast.

Cramp:

-Go to bed with 5 corks in a bag and say: *"Goodbye to cramp"*

-Or recite the following:

> *"The devil is tying a knot in my leg*
> *Mark, Luke and John, I beg*
> *Crosses three now make to ease us*
> *For the Father, Holy Ghost and Jesus"*

Croup (A respiratory condition caused by a virus which affects children. It leads to swelling inside the windpipe resulting in a barking cough):

-Drink a broth made from frogs.

-Hold a living pigeon to the throat of an afflicted child and then let the bird die of starvation – as the life of the pigeon ebbed away the child would slowly and gradually recover:

> *"The child's innocence whose breath*
> *Was purchased by the pigeon's death*
> *Who while to her sweet bosom pressed*
> *Transferred her anguish to its breast"*
> (Hackwood 1924 p.150)

Cuts:

- Rub mucus from the nose on them.

- Place a cobweb over the cut.

- Rub a tallow candle on it.

- If a cut went septic a dog would be allowed to lick it.

- Burn a piece of newspaper in the fire and when black allow it to drop onto the cut.

Diarrhoea: Drink a quarter of a cupful of milk six times a day into which nutmeg has been grated

Earache:

-Hold to the ear the centre of a boiled onion wrapped in muslin.

-Hold to the ear a bag of hot salt.

-Pour warm olive oil into the ear.

Eyes:

- For inflamed eyes wash with dew water gathered on Good Friday and preserved

- For sore eyes: Wash with cold tea.

Flatulence: Toast one or two slices of bread until burnt, then break into pieces in a bowl and cover with boiling water. When cooled: drink.

Hangover: Drink powdered snails mixed in water.

Impotence: Eat fresh carrots over a period of several months.

Indigestion: Suck a small piece of coal.

Mumps: Walk around a well three times with eyes closed and chant "*mumps go away*".

Nose Bleed: Put a cold icy key or white stone down the sufferers back.

Quinsy (An abscess between the tonsils and the wall of the throat):

-Wear around the neck a thick bandage filled with powdered resin and take two ounces of Epsom salts every morning until cured.

-Apply goose fat to throat with feather.

Rheumatism:

-Carry a powerful magnet in the pocket.

-Wear a copper ring or bracelet.

-Keep a new potato in pocket for a year.

-Place nettles under bed sheets.

-Apply to the affected area mixture of one wine glass of turpentine; two wine glasses crab apple vinegar and raw egg.

Sprains: Wear a thin strand of worsted around the affected part.

Sore Throat:

-Eat a lump of butter coated with sugar.

-Gargle with a mixture of cayenne pepper warm vinegar and boiled water.

Stiff Neck:

-A freshly removed sock was wrapped around the neck and left there overnight.

-Rub a warm iron over the neck.

Stings: Press half a raw onion to affected area for five minutes.

Stomach Ulcer: Swallow several little frogs alive.

Styes (a small, painful lump on the inside or outside of the eyelid usually caused by an eye infection known in the Black Country as a "*Powke*" as it feels like having received a poke in the eye):

- Rubbing a gold ring nine times upon it:

> *"If you rub a golden ring*
> *Upon a powke nine times*
> *The powke will surely go"*
> (Freeman 1931)

-Rub with scrap of stolen beef.

Toothache:

-Take a small piece of raw beef and press it onto the side of the face where the problem was for seven hours. As the meat decayed the toothache would subside.

-Wear the tooth of a dead man on a thread around the neck.

-Wear a mole's right or left forepaw, depending on which tooth causing pain (right for left tooth, left for right tooth).

-Toast a large cabbage leaf , wrap it in a flannel and held on the face near the aching tooth.

Warts:

-Application of water in which parings of horses hoof had been boiled.

-Similar to toothache: Take small piece of raw beef and press it onto the wart for seven hours then bury it. As the meat decayed the wart would disappear.

-As with corns: Wet them nine mornings in succession with one's own fasting spittle.

-Tie with a silken thread.

-Rub them with the tail of a tom cat in May.

-Circle seven times with right hand while looking at the at the full moon.

-Place the shape of a moon cut in an onion and say : *"New moon, true moon, take this wart away"*.

-Rub with a live snail then impale it on a thorn, (as the snail dies, the wart will disappear).

-Apply washing soda.

-Tie as many knots as possible in a piece of cotton then flush it down the toilet, but do not tell anyone about it.

-Rub the wart on the hand of a dead man.

-Rub with the sap of a dandelion stem.

A Weak Child: Taking a towel, and for nine successive mornings make it wet with May dew and with it bathe the child's body.

Whooping Cough:

-Pass the afflicted child under the branches of a common bramble bush or wild rose which has taken root at both ends, nine times on three successive mornings before sunrise while chanting the following over and over:

> *"Under the briar and over the briar*
> *I wish to leave the chin cough here"*

The briar must be cut and made into a cross and worn on the breast.

-Passing an afflicted child nine times over the back and under the belly of a donkey.

-Wearing a peppercorn necklace.

-An egg is placed in a jar and covered with vinegar until the shell dissolves, then the skin is removed and the contents, (the vinegar, white and yolk), beaten and the mixture given by spoon three times a day.

-Drinking water into which a red hot cinder had been dropped and then allowed to cool.

-Take a toad, cut off its front feet and sew them in a bag. The bag was suspended around the neck of the afflicted child and the toad set free. As it died, the cough would leave the child.

-A raw potato was suspended around the neck until it dried.

-A cure in favour in Moxley, Bilston, was to take the child along the canal side in the direction of the chemical works (this may have been due to the pungent air of the neighbourhood and the belief that the air would dispel the bad air causing the illness).

-Take the sufferer to different places for each of seven consecutive days to breathe in different airs and smells, one of which should be hot tar, (the rationale being the same as above).

-A cure popular with colliers wives was to take the sufferer down the pit.

-If a person suffering from whooping cough spat on a piece of raw meat and then fed it to a dog, the illness would be transferred to the dog.

-Take the child and allow it to see the new moon, lift up its clothes and rub your hand up and down its stomach and chest while saying:

"What I see, may it increase,
"What I feel, may it decrease
"In the name of the father, son and Holy Ghost"

-For severe cases some hair was cut from the cross on a donkey's neck and sewed up in a little silk bag which the child had to wear near to its breast.

-To make a child forever immune from the whooping cough, pass it through a large hole in the trunk of a growing tree

4 HERBAL REMEDIES

The oldest healing tradition in history is through the use of herbs or medicinal plants (Collins 2000), which formed the basis for modern pharmaceuticals. The Black Country has a strong tradition of such healing: Ogier Ward (1832) and Hackwood (1924) observed that people in the Black Country were great believers in "*Yarb Tay*" or herb tea which were infusions of herbs in hot water and it would not be unusual for most gardens to contain a few healing herbs. Chemists frequently used herbs as did Folk Healers or Charmers.

Please note: the following herbal remedies are for historical interest only. Herbal remedies should only be used following the guidance of a qualified herbalist.

Agrimony (Agrimonia Eupatoria) (aka "Sticklewort", Cockleburr"): Taken as a tea to alleviate gout and as a gargle for mouth and throat infections.

Angelica (Archangelica Officinalis): Due to the sweet scent of its root it was much valued as remedy for plague, (the sweet smell keeping away the miasma: the poisoned air which caused the plague according to contemporary beliefs); as an antidote for poison and for application to sprained limbs as a poultice[6].

Bittersweet (Solanum Dulcamara) (aka Woody Nightshade): It was believed to aid the development of clairvoyance and second sight.

Black Peppermint (Menthe Piperita): Taken as a tea used to treat colds.

Bluebell (Hyacinthoides Non-scripta): Crushed stalks were applied as a poultice for sprains.

Broom (Genisteae): A tea of the Broom flower, imbibed cold was

---

[6] Poultice: a soft, moist mass of healing material, usually herbs, applied to the body and kept in place with a cloth

used to purify the blood and as a wash to cure pimples.

Burdock (Arctium): Was useful in chronic conditions as a tea.

Chamomile (Chamaemelum Nobile): Dried "blows" or flowers were used in poultices and as a tea for people who were agitated, (Chamomile has traditionally been used as a sedative see Collins 2000).

Chickweed (Stellaria Media): Mixed with ground ivy, rose leaves, boiled water, sugar and brandy, it was a cure for weak eyes. The eyes were washed with this mixture every morning.

Coltsfoot (Tussilago Farfara)*(aka Cough Wort[7]): The flower of coltsfoot was used to brew an infusion for winter coughs, but was only effective if gathered in the spring and properly dried in paper bags hung from the kitchen ceiling through the summer months.

Comfrey (Syphytum Officinale): Leaves were applied as poultice to fractures and sprains.

Common Ivy (Hedera Helix): Itchy eyes were bathed with water in which ivy leaves had been boiled.

Cowslip (Primula Veris): Taken as a tea for headaches, insomnia and bad nerves.

Dandelion (Taraxacum Officinale): The liquid from dandelion stalks was applied to warts.

Dock Leaves (Rumex): Used to treat nettle stings.

Elderflower (Sambucus Nigra): Taken as a tea to treat colds.

Eyebright (Euphrasia *Officinalis*): Infusion used as a wash for all eye problems.

Hops (Humulus Lupulus): Used to relieve insomnia and menstrual problems.

Heather (Calluna Vulgaris): Aching feet were soaked in water, (as hot as could be tolerated), in which heather has been heated.

---

[7] Wort is a Saxon word meaning healing plant.

House Leek (Sempervivum Tectorum): A "powke" or stye and bruises were bathed with its juice.

Linseed/Flax (*Linum Usitatissimum*): Taken as a tea mixed with liquorice to treat colds.

Liverwort (Anemone Hepatica): A tea of leaves and flowers was taken as a remedy for indigestion and liver disorders.

Marsh Mallow (Althaea Officinalis): The leaves, roots and flowers were boiled in water and strained; it was good for chest problems such as coughs, Bronchitis[8] and Whooping Cough.

Mistletoe: It was customary to place mistletoe on the altar at Wolverhampton's Collegiate Church during Christmas Eve. It was then distributed among the locals who thought the blessed mistletoe possessed miraculous healing powers, especially for fevers.

Mountain Flax (Linum Cathartilum): Used as a purgative.

Mouse Ear Hawkweed (Hieracium Pilosella): Taken as a tea, sweetened with honey, for whooping cough and lung infections.

Nettle (Urtica Urens): Taken as a tea for anaemia, blood and skin disorders and urinary problems.

Parsley (Petroselinum Crispum): Taken as a tea for kidney problems.

Raspberry (Rubus Idaeus): The leaves, taken as a tea, eased pregnancy and with blackcurrant leaves, cloves and cinnamon for fevers.

Solomon's Seal (Polygonatum Multiflorum): Ointment made from the leaves was used to treat baldness and bruises.

Valerian (Valeriana Officnales): The juice of a fresh root was used to treat epilepsy and hysteria. Valerian has traditionally been used as a sedative (Collins 2000)

Watercress (Nasturtium Officinale): Taken as a tea as a cure for Whooping Cough.

---

[8] Bronchitis: An inflammation of the mucous membrane in the bronchial tubes

White Horehound (Marrubium Vulgare): Taken for chest complaints.

Yarrow (Achillea Millefolium): Taken as a tea, hot or cold, for colds.

There were herb shops in most Black Country towns. As already observed: Nathaniel Catlin, Quack Doctor of Bilston market, eventually opened a Herb shop on Bilston High Street. One of the most renowned shops was Denton's at Holloway End, Amblecote. It was run by George Denton, known as *'Diddy Denton the Pill Mon'*. He was a former Iron Turner who endeavoured to better himself by studying herbalism, he eventually became a member of the "National Association of Medical Herbalists of Great Britain".

AFTERWORD

Today, it is easy to deride the folk cures and beliefs of the past, secure in the faith placed in modern medicine. Yet some infections (pneumonia, tuberculosis and gonorrhoea) have become resistant to antibiotics and antibiotic resistance is considered to be one of the biggest threats to global health today by the World Health Organisation (2016). Further, modern society still has its own version of folk healing in the variety of alternative treatments available: Crystal healing; Magnet Therapy; Spiritual healing; Reiki and Homeopathy among others. Such therapies, while having their proponents, have no scientific support for their healing abilities.

The more things change: the more they stay the same.

BIBLIOGRAPHY AND REFERENCES

Bliss, E. (2014) On Immunity: An Inoculation. Graywolf Press.

Brimble, J. (1986) *Pills and Potions: Folk Medicine in the Black Country*. Black Country Society.

Collins, M. (2000) *Medieval Herbals: The Illustrative Traditions* (British Library Studies in Medieval Culture). University of Toronto Press.

Freeman, J. (1931) *Black Country Stories and Sketches*: James Wilkes: Bilston.

Hackwood, F.W. (1924) *Staffordshire Customs, Superstitions and Folklore*. E.P.Publishing: Yorkshire

Humphries, R. *It Seems Like Yesterday*. (accessed23/2/2017):http://www.blackcountrymemories.org.uk/pages1/humphries.htm

Mnookin, S.(2012) The Panic Virus: The True Story Behind the Vaccine-Autism Controversy. Simon & Schuster.

Ogier Ward, T. (1834)"Observations upon Cholera" *Transactions of the Provincial Medical and Surgical Association* 1844-48, 370-90

Palmer, R. (2007) *The Folklore of the Black Country*. Logaston Press,

Parkes, J. (1915) *A History of Tipton*. Elton and Brown. Tipton.

Poland, G.A. (2011) MMR Vaccine and Autism: Vaccine Nihilism and Postmodern Science *Mayo Clinic Proceedings, 86(9)*: 869–871.

Poole, C.H. (1875) The *Customs, Superstitions and Legends of the County of Stafford*. London: Rowney and co.

Porter, R. (2003) *Quacks: Fakers & Charlatans in Medicine*. Tempus.

Raven, J. (1986) Stories, Customs, Superstitions, Tales, Legends and Folklore of the Black Country and Staffordshire. Wolverhampton: Broadside.

Report and Appendices of the Children's Employment Commission. Presented to both Houses of Parliament, by Command of her Majesty. *The Monthly Review* . April 1843.

Soloman, P. (1992) Black Country Ways In Bygone Days. Willenhall: PKN Publications

The Condition and Treatment of the Children Employed In the Mines and Collieries of the United Kingdom (1842). London: William Strange.

Walsall Local History Centre (1992) *I Remember Walsall Market.* Oral History from Walsall Local History Centre.

White, W. (1860) "All round the Wrekin". Chapman and Hall: London.

World Health Organisation (October 2016) Fact Sheet: *Antibiotic Resistance*(Accessed:29/2/2017):

http://www.who.int/mediacentre/factsheets/antibiotic-resistance/en/

Printed in Great Britain
by Amazon

84759668R00031